Explo

A ruptured cerebral aneurysm and
subarachnoid haemorrhage;

a survivor's story

Anne Reavill

Contents

Prologue

There are innumerable accounts relating the experiences of those who have suffered life threatening illness, now told in books or blogs. Many people find the process of writing therapeutic, especially where their treatment and (hopefully) recovery was long drawn out. I never thought I would be one of them, and initially had no inclination to record my own experience, feeling that writing about it would be rather self indulgent. But any serious illness is highly traumatic, both for the sufferers and those near to them. Three and a half years elapsed before I started to write and during this time never a day has gone by when I have not thought and sometimes even dreamt about what happened, although looking back now it often all seems unreal. I am lucky in that I have recovered so well with no serious side effects as reminders.

I had a stroke, but not the usual kind. Most strokes are caused by ischaemic attacks, where the blood supply to part of the brain in severely reduced or cut off completely. This leads to damage of the brain cells in that region, with correspondingly serious consequences. However a few percent of strokes are different. They are due to what is known as a subarachnoid haemorrhage, usually caused, as in my case, by a ruptured cerebral aneurysm.

A subarachnoid haemorrhage is a bleed into the space surrounding the brain, not into the brain tissue itself. The brain and spinal cord are surrounded by a liquid, the cerebrospinal fluid, and this fills the subarachnoid space. This fluid, amongst other things, acts as a buffer, helping to protect the brain from injury during sudden movement or a blow to the head. More detailed anatomy shows that this space is bounded by two membranes, below is the pia mater, the membrane covering the brain, and above it attached indirectly to the skull is the arachnoid membrane. The arachnoid membrane and pia mater are attached by fine strands spanning the subarachnoid space and between which the cerebrospinal fluid flows.

Blood vessels, which enter the subarachnoid space, snake and branch out over the surface of the brain, delivering necessary nutrients and removing waste products. Occasionally an aneurysm forms on one of these vessels, often at the junctions where they branch into two. They develop where there is a weakness in the arterial wall, causing it first to distend and then go on to form a sac like structure, usually with a narrow neck. As blood is pumped along the artery, it is forced into the aneurysm and the pressure can eventually lead to its rupture. Unless they bleed an aneurysm is usually symptomless and many people never know they have one. They go on to live a normal life span and die of something quite unrelated. But sometimes, without any warning, they burst, resulting in a subarachnoid haemorrhage.

With a large volume of blood entering the subarachnoid space, pressure increases dramatically, and bleeding may only cease when pressure equals that in the blood vessels. It is this pressure on the brain that is the cause of the severe headache. The sudden headache has been likened to a thunderclap and described as the worst headache ever. Blood itself is also highly irritant to brain cells, and this can go on to cause further problems.

When the bleed is severe death can be instantaneous, and it has been estimated that between 30 - 40 % of people who suffer a subarachnoid haemorrhage die either immediately or very soon afterwards. Around another 30% will be left with moderate to severe brain damage and the remainder may have no more than slight damage or even make a complete recovery. This, then, is my own story, recounting what I remember of the acute stage, surgery, time in intensive care, and slow recovery, first in hospital and then at home over the following months and years.

1

The explosions

There are no warning signs. Today has been an ordinary one, and I have not done anything unusual or stressful. With me and my husband both retired from full time work we now have time to enjoy life. We are fit and active and, amongst other things, are regular walkers, sometimes gently along the Thames Path and more energetically up and along the Ridgeway Path. Tonight we are on our way to bed. I have washed, brushed my teeth and am almost ready to get into bed. Lawrie is in the bathroom. We have no idea of the time bomb about to go off.

I run a comb through my hair, and am suddenly aware of a sound within my head, a loud, regular beat—my heart beat? But surely I shouldn't be able to hear it like that, so loud. It quickly fades and disappears.

I stand and think. What on earth was that? Surely that is not normal. Could it be something serious? I am worried. What should I do?

I could phone the doctor on call on the out of hour's advice line. But what would I say?

All I could tell them was that briefly I had heard a loud thumping beat in my head, it has now stopped and I feel perfectly alright. They would probably just say to wait and see, and call them if it happened again or got worse. So perhaps that is what I should do.

I decide to wait and see, so carry on tidying away my clothes and a minute or two later get into bed.

As I lie down it starts again. This is not right, I think. I am definitely going to phone the duty doctor.

But this time the beating does not stop. It gets louder and hard, each one an explosion—bang—bang—bang .....

It is like having my head hit hard against a brick wall.

Bang—bang—bang ..... Will it ever stop? It goes on and on.

Then suddenly—silence.

Thank goodness.

But my relief is short lived. The next moment I am suffocating. I can't get my breath. I am panicking. I am breathing as hard as I can and throw my arms up above my head in an attempt to get more air in my lungs.

Then I am aware of another soft thump, a pause, and then another, not as loud and hard as before. My heart must be beating, but too slowly I think, and, as the rate increases, I can get my breath again. Now the beating fades.

It is over.

I am lying feeling stunned. I know it must be a stroke. My first thoughts—am I paralysed? You hear of people being completely paralysed after strokes— a nightmare. But I can move. To my relief I feel I can move my toes, although am too weak to do any more than that. Where is Lawrie? I need help. It is no use calling; his hearing is not good. But there is no way I can get to him. I have to wait. I am willing him to come soon.

It seems an age, but is probably no more than a couple of minutes until he finishes his wash and brushing of teeth and returns to the bedroom. He starts to get into bed.

Can I speak? 'Lawrie,' I manage to get the words out. 'Something's happened in my head. I need help.'

He does not hear me properly as I can only speak softly.

'You've got a headache? Do you want some aspirin?'

'No! It's serious. I need a doctor.'

He jumps back out of bed.

'I'll phone.'

I hear him talking to someone on the phone, though not what is being said. He comes back to me, but before he can say anything, without any warning, I find I am being sick. I want to grab something to be sick into, but can't move as the vomit runs round my neck and into the bed. Lawrie comes to me and wipes it away as best he can with some tissues.

The phone rings and Lawrie speaks briefly to someone, then to me.

'They're sending an ambulance.'

Thank goodness. Help is coming. I can relax.

Then I am sick again.....

* * *

'Mrs Reavill.'

I hear the voice and open my eyes for a moment to see someone standing beside my bed.

'Mrs Reavill, I'm Doctor.....' I immediately forget his name.

I am in hospital and remember what has happened. I listen to what the doctor is telling me. I have had a bleed into the space around my brain due to a ruptured aneurysm. I must have had a scan, I think to myself. (I have had a CT scan and this revealed a large subarachnoid haemorrhage.

I cannot remember anything about having this done, or indeed of my journey to the Royal Berkshire Hospital in Reading.) The doctor goes on to explain more, but I already know.

I have to tell him. I manage to get the words out.

'My mother had that.'

'So you know about what it is?'

'Yes.'

'So the question now is what to do about it.'

I will have to have an operation, I think to myself. The aneurysm will have to be sealed off so it cannot bleed again. But what he says surprises me. He explains that it is sometimes possible to run a catheter via the artery in my groin up to my brain and to the aneurysm. Then very small coils of platinum wire can be inserted into the sac of the aneurysm. This causes blood to clot within the sac and eventually it closes off completely.

I have never heard of this procedure. It sounds wonderful—so much better than the sort of brain surgery I had been imagining. Things have progresses considerably since my mother's day.

'Unfortunately we don't do that sort of thing here,' the doctor goes on. 'So I'm going to contact the Neuroscience Unit at the John Radcliffe Hospital in Oxford and see if we can transfer you there. Is that OK?'

'Yes. Thank you.'

I am vaguely aware of Lawrie with me, holding my hand.

* * *

My mother

My mother died in 1974. A year or so earlier she had been shopping in Torquay where she and my father lived. She was in a department store with a friend when suddenly she had an intense pain in her head. Someone found her a chair to sit on as she vomited back her lunch. She had a terrible headache and her friend took her home.

My father called a GP who came and examined her. She still had a bad headache and neck stiffness. He told her she had pulled a muscle in her back and the pain was referred to her head and neck!

I was away working as a midwife near London and only got a letter from my father telling me she had been unwell several days later. I was home a few days after that, by which time she appeared fully recovered. She had spent several days in bed and she described her symptoms to me. She had had

14

a persistent dreadful headache. Some children outside had been playing with a ball, kicking it against a wall, and the noise had been almost unbearable. She had not been able to stand light and had kept her curtains drawn all the time.

I was horrified. This was supposed to be due to a pulled muscle in her back? I couldn't believe a doctor would have thought this. Being a nurse I recognized these as cerebral symptoms. Later I discussed this with one of my aunts, who had also been a nurse, and she thought the same as me. But what could I do now? I didn't want to alarm or frighten my parents, and my mother appeared to have fully recovered, so I decided not to say anything. But if anything like it ever happened again I was going to make certain it was investigated properly in hospital.

A year or so later my parents were staying with my sister and her family in Australia. They were all out together one evening when my mother suddenly collapsed with similar symptoms, headache and vomiting. This time she was taken to hospital, where she seemed to recover quickly and they sent her home after a day or two. But exactly a week later she collapsed again and this time became and remained unconscious. In hospital they did eventually do an angiogram, which revealed the aneurysm. They started talking about surgery, but a day later she suffered another bleed, her condition deteriorated rapidly and she died.

At the time I felt like blaming the GP who said that her first attack was due to pulling a muscle in her back, but I am not sure that, even if she had been sent to hospital, it would have made any difference in the end. This was the early seventies when things were very different to now. The sort of scans we can do today were not available and the usual way to diagnose a subarachnoid haemorrhage was by doing a lumbar puncture, which would show blood in the cerebrospinal fluid, but does not reveal the cause or location of an aneurysm. Even so in many cases no further treatment would be given. The only available treatment then was clipping which, even when possible, was a major operation, and the risks of neurosurgery were then often considered too great. Today clipping is still a major operation, hence the procedure of inserting wire coils, known as endovascular coiling, is the treatment of choice.

* * *

Oxford

'The ambulance is here. We are going to move you now.'

It is a woman's voice. A nurse probably. I am rolled to one side and then back onto something hard and flat, then slid across this onto a trolley.

* * *

I am in the ambulance. I open my eyes and look around, suddenly feeling wide awake. I look at the windows and can see silhouettes of trees passing against a faint glow of sky. It must be morning. (I later find out it is after midday and the reason it does not appear fully light is because the glass in the ambulance's windows is heavily tinted.)

I hope we get there soon.....

* * *

There are several people around me. 'I am going to put in a catheter,' someone is saying.

A catheter? For a moment I wonder why I should need one, but then realise it is a good idea. I cannot move to get to the toilet and it will mean I don't have to use an uncomfortable bedpan either.....

* * *

I am in a room on my own. I try to look around. Where is Lawrie? He must have gone somewhere. I am sure he will be back soon.

Someone has come to do my recordings. She attaches the blood pressure cuff and I feel it pump up and then slowly release. She flashes a light into each of my eyes in turn, checking that my pupils react equally.....

* * *

Lawrie is with me again now and I feel reassured by his presence. (Later he tells me that there was no room for him to come with me in the ambulance because there was only a small one available. He had to make his way home, where he was able to catch up with a wash and change, and then follow me to Oxford in the car. He must have been so tired, having been with me all night at the hospital in Reading.)

* * *

Someone is taking my recordings again. Lawrie says goodbye and leaves me to go home and I am settled for the night. Apart from feeling extremely weak and drowsy I don't feel ill; don't even have a headache, although my eyes hurt when I move them. For a short while I lie awake, wondering what is going to happen. Perhaps they will decide in the morning. (I am quite unaware that I have had a CT angiogram that afternoon. The scan shows I have had a large bleed and have a right inferior frontal clot. It is rated as 4 on the Fisher scale of 1-4. It also revealed the location and size of the aneurysm. It measures 5x3 mm and is described as a tri-lobed left A1/2 junction aneurysm. I can remember nothing of the procedure.) Strangely, although there have been long stretches of time where I can remember nothing of what has happened, I have never woken wondering where I am.

I do know, however, that an aneurysm can bleed again at any time. As well as my mother I know of two other people who died from this same condition. One was a nurse in a hospital I was working in. She was on duty on the ward when she suddenly collapsed and died immediately. I did not know her personally, but was still shocked at the time. The other was the father of someone I used to work with. He collapsed one evening and was taken into hospital where he died during the night.

I am thinking of them all now, but in spite of this I am not really afraid. I tell myself that I could die at any moment, and yet it all seems unreal. I am tired, so don't think about it anymore; just sleep.

* * *

It is morning. A group of doctors come into my room. They introduce themselves but once again I instantly forget their names.

'I understand your mother had an aneurysm,' one of them says to me.

'Yes. She died.'

'So you know how serious it is.'

I nod.

'Well we don't think we can leave it any longer. There is the danger it will bleed again. It could happen at any time, so we need to do something now.'

He explains to me again about the operation, endovascular coiling it is called. It will have to be done under a general anaesthetic, not because it is painful but because they have to be certain that I keep absolutely still during the procedure. Even the slightest movement could result in serious damage, possibly rupturing the aneurysm. He also tells me of the success rate of the operation and the possible complications, as he is obliged to do. These include another bleed or a stroke. But the dangers of leaving it are much greater.

'What about your husband?' he then asks. 'He should know what we are going to do. Would you like me to call him?'

I say that I would.

He goes to make the call. (He explains everything in detail to Lawrie and asks him if he is happy for them to proceed. He tells them he is happy if I am.)

He returns and tells me he has contacted Lawrie and explained it all to him. If I am agreeable they will do the operation now. I say that I am.

'Can you manage to sign the consent form?' He has it there ready.

I am not sure that I can. It takes a supreme effort to lift my arm. A pen is put into my hand.

'Where do I sign?'

You should always read things before signing, but I don't have my glasses and have no idea where they are—at home probably. But I trust them implicitly. The doctor indicates where I should sign and I manage a signature of sorts. They all then leave saying they will be ready for me very shortly.

I am just thankful that something is being done. I lie there thinking, but not for long. The theatre trolley arrives.

It all still seems unreal. I am not worried or afraid and have complete faith in everyone. I am going to be alright. I have to think that. In the theatre anaesthetic room I stare at the ceiling as the anaesthetist starts to inject something into the cannula in the back of my hand.....

* * *

Endovascular coiling.

As I have mentioned, endovascular coiling involves inserting a fine tube into the femoral artery in the groin from where it is navigating up through the arteries to the brain and the tip guided into the aneurysm. Once there, minute coils of platinum wire are threaded up through the tube and gently inserted into the aneurysm. Within the aneurysm the coils interrupt the flow of blood so that it clots within the coils. Eventually no further blood can enter and the aneurysm will become completely sealed off.

Endovascular coiling was developed in the nineteen nineties. Before that, as in my mother's day, the only option for sealing an aneurysm was to clip it off. This is a much more invasive procedure as it involves a craniotomy, where a small flap of bone from the skull is removed in order to get direct access to the brain, a procedure which has additional risks, such as bleeding and infection. However not all aneurysms can be treated this way; some are just too difficult or dangerous to access. Nowadays these can often be treated by coiling.

The main disadvantage of coiling is that in a small proportion of cases it is not totally successful. Sometimes the coils bed down and the procedure needs to be repeated to add more, and very occasionally the aneurysm will still need clipping to seal it off completely. However today coiling is the treatment of choice where possible and this is what I am having done.

2

Intensive care

I am back in my room. One of the doctors is with me and asks how I am feeling. I say I am alright. She tells me the operation went well and I have had three platinum coils successfully implanted into the aneurysm. Then she examines me to make sure I am not developing any side effect from the operation. She sees that I can lift each of my legs equally and then gets me to hold her fingers so she can compare the strength of my grip in either hand. This is to ensure that there is no weakness developing on either side, possible first signs of a stroke. My pupil reactions are checked and then I am asked a couple of simple questions, like 'what year is it?' and 'who is the prime minister?', to make sure I am not becoming mentally confused. I soon become used to these neurological tests as the nurses repeat them at regular intervals throughout the coming days. Now I don't feel any different from before except that my back is aching, as it often does if I lie flat for too long. It is making me restless. I want to sit up.

'You mustn't sit up yet,' the doctor says. 'You need to try to relax. Remember you have had neurosurgery, even if it doesn't feel like it.'

Later I have some painkillers for my backache and am more settled. Surprisingly I don't have a headache and it is hard to believe I have had anything done to me at all, let alone neurosurgery.

Lawrie is with me again. He tells me he has contacted my sister in Australia to let her know of my illness and they have talked on the phone. He has also brought in a few of my wash things, which he puts into my locker, then stays sitting at the bedside as I dose on and off.

I am awakened by the loud roar of an approaching engine. Lawrie goes to the window and looks out.

'It's a helicopter. The landing site is just outside here. They must be bringing someone in.' I would like to look, but am too far from the window.

A nurse comes in with more pills. The important one is nimodipine, I have been told. Nimodipine is an antihypertensive drug which specifically reduces pressure in the blood vessels of the brain. This reduces the risk of developing vasospasm in these vessels, a serious complication that can occur after a subarachnoid haemorrhage and which can lead to serious brain damage, even death. Blood vessels in the brain go into spasm, contracting so as to reduce or cut off the circulation to part of the brain. The result is similar to that of a stroke. It can develop several days after the initial haemorrhage, most commonly in the first three weeks, peaking after three or four days I am told. They need to remain vigilant in watching for signs that it might be developing; hence the frequent neurological tests carried out by the nurses. I will have to continue taking nimodipine for three weeks to reduce the chances of developing vasospasm.

I awake early the following morning and lie staring at the ceiling, which I am beginning to know well by now. It is covered in plain white square tiles, each measuring around half a metre across. But today it looks different; the lines won't come together. I have double vision.

A nurse comes in to do my recordings, all normal, but when she goes on to do my neurological examination I find it harder to move my legs. Then I am given a pot containing several pills to take and a cup of tea in a feeding mug, most of which I manage to drink.

The doctors come in to see me on their morning rounds and ask how I am feeling.

'I've got double vision.'

They look a bit concerned and continue to ponder over my notes. The double vision together with my worsening leg weakness are probable signs of vasospasm. One of them suggests an MRI scan, but I cannot have that done because I have a pacemaker. (The high magnetic fields generated by these scans will damage a pacemaker.) They leave the room. A short while later one of them returns.

'You seem to be doing well, but I think to be on the safe side we need to keep a much closer eye on you. We want to move you to the intensive care unit where we can do that more easily. As I say, this is mainly a precaution.'

He does not want to worry me too much. Almost immediately after that I am wheeled on my bed down to the Neuroscience Intensive Care Unit on the floor below. There I am slid across onto a new bed. I am already feeling cold and this makes me feel even colder. I pull my covers up over me.

I now have one nurse looking after me and she carries out the usual observations. Her presence is reassuring.

'Are you feeling cold?' she asks, probably seeing me shivering.

'Yes.'

'I can get you an electric blanket. Would like that?'

An electric blanket? I didn't know they had such things in hospitals. In my imagination I visualise the sort of blankets we used to have in my childhood that went under the bottom sheet and were used to warm beds before getting in. But this one turns out to be very different.

She puts the blanket over my top sheet and attaches it to a machine that blows it up with warm air. It expands and folds itself over me, and is absolute bliss.

'That's wonderful.' I say, instantly feeling better.

Like all patients in hospital today I am wearing anti-DVT socks. These are tight, knee length socks with a bit that can fold back at the end so you can get to the toes if needed. DVT, or deep vein thrombosis to give it its full name, is where the blood clots within the leg veins. It can happen during a long period of inactivity because blood is circulating more slowly than usual, giving it time to start clotting. The danger is that the clot then becomes loose or a piece breaks off and moves through the circulation to become lodged in the lungs or brain even. If this happens it can be fatal. Now, as an additional precaution, I have cuffs over the socks round each of my calves, and these are attached to a machine which blows up and releases each in turn. This makes them contract and relax rhythmically on alternate legs. As I am hardly moving at all this is helping to keep my circulation going and prevent blood from clotting in the veins.

I am in a corner of the unit. To my right is a curtain partially drawn across with what looks like various bits of equipment beyond, and to my left there is my locker and a chair between my bed and the wall. A bit further ahead the ward extends round a corner to the left. In the distance opposite I can see windows, but I cannot see any of the other patients since all beds seem to be surrounded by equipment. It is very quiet, just the hum of machinery and occasional bleeping of monitors. My nurse stands by my locker writing in my notes and a couple of others come to join her for a while, probably to see what is going on with me, and they talk quietly. It all seems very calm and unhurried.

Someone comes to take a blood sample, which I seem to be having taken at least once a day. Later I am told that my potassium levels are low and my nurse brings me some revolting tasting liquid to drink to boost levels. I get Lawrie to bring me in some bananas, which I know are high in potassium. I have eaten nothing for the last two days, but now light meals are brought to me and I am managing to eat a little. Although I am drinking a bit, I still have my drip going to keep up my fluid intake. I seem to be surrounded by tubes of one kind or another; the drip, catheter, and a probe inserted into my femoral artery on the opposite side from where the tube had been inserted for the endovascular coiling. This probe had been used during my operation to measure arterial blood pressure directly; far more accurate than using the usual blood pressure machine (sphygmomanometer) that records it from your arm.

Visiting hours are more flexible here, and Lawrie can come in at more or less any time of the day. Also, because I am in intensive care, he has been given a free pass for the car park, which is very useful. It must be very boring for him, as most of the time I just dose off. I don't seem to be able to keep awake for very long at any one time. He usually stays for a while, then goes off to a nearby pub that serves bar food, then back to visit me for bit longer. He has brought me in a beautifully scented single rose from the garden, which he places in a small container on my locker. I am not sure that we are supposed to have flowers in here, but no one removes it.

I am brought a small pot with around half a dozen pills to take at regular intervals These include the nimodipine, although on a couple of occasions they have to halve the dose to one tablet because my blood pressure is too low. Although it works mainly on blood vessels in the brain, nimodipine does also reduce the general blood pressure a bit. My blood pressure is usually normal and can be a bit low at times, so they do not want it to drop too much more. My temperature is up a bit and, after listening to my chest, they think I am developing a chest infection, so I start a course of antibiotics. I am also given painkillers, either paracetamol or codeine, which I am taking more for backache than headache, plus some very sickly sweet liquid for my bowels, which have become extremely sluggish; not surprising seeing I have eaten virtually nothing. I also need to continue the liquid potassium for a few days until my blood levels are normal.

There is nothing for me to do, but all I want is to doze anyway. When awake I gaze at the ceiling, which has the same white squares as the room I was in before. When I look to the right the lines come together, but the further I move my eyes to the left, the more they separate again. I concentrate on trying to get the lines closer, at least when I look straight ahead. Double vision is a common after effect of a subarachnoid haemorrhage. If I want to read I have been told that I may find it easier if I cover one eye. However I am far from wanting to read anything at the moment, and I don't know where my glasses are anyway. I persevere and by the end of the week the degree of my double vision is definitely reduced, so I am confident that in time it will resolve completely.

After my first couple of days in intensive care I am no longer considered one of their most acutely ill and start sharing my nurse with another patient. I now tend to have someone different most days, although the one at night is almost always the same, a cheerful young nurse.

I have been in bed for almost a week before I get out for the first time. I take it very slowly with two nurses helping. First both legs over the side and then slide forward until my feet are on the floor. But I cannot take my weight and am more or less lifted over to the chair. I can't believe how weak I have become.

'Well you have been in bed for almost a week,' Lawrie says to me when I worry about this.

'But surely I shouldn't be this helpless?'

I am told I must give it time.

The next day I am given my early morning tea. It is still a bit hot, so I hold it, resting on my bed beside me. The next thing I am aware of is a warm, wet feeling down my side—the tea. I have dozed off again and it has spilt in my bed. I call to my nurse.

'I'm so sorry. I just fell asleep again. The bed is soaked.'

She takes it all in her stride. Someone comes to help and my bed is changed.

Later I hear another patient kicking up a fuss.

'I'm going home,' she is shouting. 'I've had enough. I don't want to stay here.'

The nurses try to placate her, but she gets more agitated and confused.

'Don't, you mustn't pull that out. You will bleed.' One of the nurses, must be trying to restrain her from trying to remove one of her tubes.

This goes on for several minutes, but eventually the woman calms down. It is the only time I hear anything from another patient while I am here.

I do not develop any more symptoms and it seems that the serious consequences of vasospasm have been averted. Although still weak I am able to move my legs normally once again and my double vision is resolving. I have been here almost a week when the doctors say I am well enough to return to the ward. I am wheeled back, once again to a single room. I am making progress.

3

The danger period

I have been told I will need to stay in hospital for a total of three weeks following on from the time of the operation. This is what they refer to as the 'danger period' when the risk of bleeding again is highest. The risk of bleeding following a subarachnoid haemorrhage is highest within the first two days and then peaks again at between 7-10 days. I have survived over a week now, so soon the danger will soon start to diminish. In my new room the nurses come to do my observations every four hours, staff bring my meals and I still seem to have to take a lot of pills. From time to time I see people go by my open door, otherwise it is very quiet. However I do not stay there for long. A couple of days later I am moved to a four bedded ward, and to the beginning of what in many ways I find to be the hardest time of my stay in hospital.

My bed is wheeled into place next to the window and, once settled, I manage to say hello to my three roommates. They don't say much and I find trying to speak at all is a great effort, so I just doze off again.

From overhearing conversations on my first day, I discover one of the others has had the same as me. I would like to talk to her, but don't have the energy to try to speak to someone in the far corner from me and I am unable to go over to her. The next day she goes home, so I miss my chance. Her place is soon taken by someone else.

Lawrie is here to visit every day. When he first arrives he tells me the news from home and brings in my post, if there is any. I then open my post, and most goes straight in the bin as usual. After that I am exhausted and dose off for a bit. Lawrie is used to me dozing off while he is there and always brings something with him to read. Then it is supper time. Every morning a menu is brought round and I spend time studying it and making my selection. I have now found my glasses so I can see to read again. Eating is such an effort that I don't manage too much anyway. Lawrie tries to encourage me and in the end often starts to feed me himself. I feel I am being very lazy but at the same time I find it really soothing to be fed like this. I can take my time, resting between mouthfuls, and do manage to eat more this way.

The other patients often complain about the food, but most of what they have suits me. I stick things like lasagne or cauliflower cheese, which are light and easy to eat. The only other thing I feel I would like is fish. At one time steamed fish was a basic constituent of an invalid diet, but it seems no longer so. There is grilled fish one day, which I try, but it is rather dry and I do not enjoy it much. That is the only time I see it on the menu. Perhaps fish is too expensive for hospitals today.

Every few days Lawrie brings me a fresh rose from the garden, as he started doing when I was in ICU. They are blooming well at the moment and are all beautifully scented varieties—not planted by us but by the previous occupants of our house.

'You're not supposed to have flowers here. They can be a source of infection,' a nurse tells us on more than one occasion, but no attempts are made to remove it. I never have more than one at a time in a small container, a new one simply replacing one that is fading.

Like all patients, I have an allocated nurse every day, but most days it is somebody different and I see very little of them now, usually just when they first come on duty and then when they hand out pills at the appropriate times. Only one nurse seems to have this room assigned to her regularly. She is young and efficient in her work, but like all of them always seem busy and does not have time to chat. A health care assistance does most of the routine observations and the frequency of my neurological tests are reduced.

Up until now Lawrie has been my only visitor. Even with him I can only talk for a few minutes before having to rest. He is used to this now, but I don't feel up to talking to anyone else, so he is putting off anybody who wants to come to visit. It is quite a distance for them to travel anyway. One of my friends does eventually come for a short visit and I enjoy seeing her again. Another day my sister phones me from Australia. Lawrie has arranged the time she should call, so I have my mobile on and ready at hand. It is good to hear from her. She has been so worried about me and was on the verge of coming all the way over here when I first became ill. Thankfully I am now recovering, albeit slowly, so there is no urgency for her to come and she is planning to visit at a later date when I am better and we can do things together.

One problem we have is the holidays we have booked. Now we have more time to ourselves we are trying to spend more of it travelling and visiting some of the places we have always wanted to go, and this year we had three holidays booked. Last week we were supposed to have been going on Eurostar to France for few days, but of course this has already been cancelled. It is almost a month until our next planned trip, this time a short cruise over to Ireland. That should be very restful, so I am sure I will be well enough to manage it by then. Lawrie is not so sure, but just says we will have to wait and see.

My recovery is frustratingly slow. I start by sitting out in a chair, but find I cannot tolerate it for long. I soon need to lie down again. However I am able to stand, if only when holding on to something. Then I take my first few steps, supported by two nurses, one on either side and one of them carrying my urinary drainage bag. The trouble I now find is that, as well as being generally unsteady, my balance will suddenly go, with me lurching mainly to my left.

The next day my catheter is removed. It has been in for two weeks and now I will have to start getting up to go to the bathroom. I am told to ring my bell when I want to go so that someone can help me. I still have a drip, so it either needs to be temporarily disconnected or my drip stand has to be wheeled with me. The first couple of times someone comes to help me on my way, but the trouble with being in a room of convalescent patients, we don't see much of the staff, who are kept busy elsewhere with the more acutely ill, (and paperwork no doubt). There can be quite a wait before anyone is able to answer a bell, and then it always seems to be answered by someone different, usually someone I have never met before. So the next time I decide I can manage on my own. I hold onto my drip stand for support and wheel it in front of me to get to the bathroom. It feels quite an achievement.

Then at last I am able to have a shower. At first I think I cannot manage as I am still unable to keep my balance when standing without holding on firmly to something. A young nurse, I think maybe a student on placement, is with me and shows me how to pull out a seat so I can sit down. I turn on the shower. It feels wonderful; my first shower for over two weeks.

After this for the first time since coming here I get out my makeup bag, which Lawrie brought in for me a while ago along with my other things. I look at myself in the mirror. I look awful, pale and drawn, and my hair, which had been due to be cut at the time I came into hospital, is now straggling almost down to my shoulders. I start with the tweezers, tidying my eyebrows a bit and removing unwanted hairs that have sprung up over the last two and a half weeks. Then a little foundation and smudge of eye shadow. I have never been one for much makeup, but think I look a bit better now for when Lawrie arrives. It seems strange to do this after so long. It is not that I have forgotten how to do it, but it is like remembering something again from long ago. I am to get this feeling many times over the next few weeks.

My double vision has almost completely resolved itself, except for when I turn my eyes over to the left. When lying in bed I don't like the light from the window and have been keeping the curtain partially drawn. Brain trauma often leads to photophobia so it might be partly this, but I have never been very tolerant of bright lights even before this happened. When Lawrie visits I get up to demonstrate my walking ability and for the first time gaze out of the window from where there is an extensive view over towards the city. I look for the helicopter pad, but it is not visible from here. The single room that I was in earlier had been facing a different direction. But I have difficulty focusing clearly. Within the ward I am alright, but my far distant vision is not so good.

As a change, with me holding onto Lawrie's arm, we go out of the room and I look down the long ward corridor. Walking is relieving my backache, which still bothers me much of the time when I lie down. The ward is extremely large; over 80 beds, I discover later, and I wonder whether to go further, but one of the nurses sees us.

'You mustn't go far from your room,' she tells me. 'Remember you are still within the danger period.'

So we just cross the corridor and briefly inspect the notice board opposite, where I do not find anything to interest me.

Although I am making progress, I get the feeling that more is expected of me. Staff encourage me to sit out of bed, and I do try, but after a few minutes I start to feel awful and just have to lie down again. I have my drip removed and am told I must drink a lot. It is especially important for my recovery to keep well hydrated. However I find this extremely difficult. Just water makes me nauseated, I can't face coffee and can only manage so much weak tea, so over the next couple of days Lawrie brings in a variety of fruit juices, bitter lemon and tonic water. This helps, but I am told I am still not drinking enough and my drip is replaced. I feel depressed about this, but at least I don't have to force myself to drink all the time.

I am beginning to feel nauseated quite a lot of the time and the doctor writes me up for something to help. Mainly, though, I find just eating is more beneficial. I feel worst before meals and the nausea is relieved by eating. The trouble I now find is that meals in hospital are not evenly spaced. Lunch is at around midday and supper barely six hours later, then nothing but a drink in the evening and a light breakfast the next morning of just cereal and toast. I start ordering more food and hording some of it for late evening and when I wake at night. As a result my locker is littered with packets of biscuits and cheese and dishes with cold deserts saved from supper.

I think the medical staff are a bit concerned by my slow progress and I have another brain scan, which shows nothing new. They next decide to do a lumbar puncture to check my intracranial pressure. One serious complication of a subarachnoid haemorrhage is a build-up of cerebrospinal fluid causing pressure on the brain, a condition known as hydrocephalus. Cerebrospinal fluid is constantly being formed in the brain, circulating around both brain and spinal cord to supply nutrients and remove waste products, and then reabsorbed into the blood stream. Sometimes after a subarachnoid haemorrhage the rate of absorption becomes reduced leading to a build-up of cerebrospinal fluid and a subsequent increase in intracranial pressure. If this happens a stent may need to be inserted to drain excess fluid away. Like vasospasm the peak incidence is between 7-10 days after a subarachnoid haemorrhage.

The lumbar puncture is quite painless. The doctor chats to me while he carries out the procedure, and this helps to take my mind off what he is doing, although I don't think I am very responsive. I lie curled on my side as he feels down my spine to select the site where he will insert the needle. He injects some local anaesthetic into the spot and then a longer needle is inserted between the vertebrae in my lower spine. Once the end of the needle is in the space surrounding the spinal cord, cerebrospinal fluid flows back under pressure, and this pressure is measured. My pressure levels are only very slightly raised, so he withdraws just a few millilitres of fluid to reduce it and am told everything is fine. Once he has removed the needle and applied a small dressing I am told to stay lying down for the next hour or so and to call someone to make sure I am alright the first time I get up afterwards. I have no after effects.

One thing the doctors always ask me when they come to see me on their morning rounds is, do I have any tingling or pins and needles in my feet or hands. I always say no, but lying there now I realize that I do feel some tingling in my feet. Up until now I have dismissed it as due to my tight anti-DVT socks, but now I am beginning to wonder. I mention it the next time they ask, but they do not seem concerned.

I never really get to know the other women in the room with me. One of them seems to have a large, extended family who are always ready waiting to come in as soon as visiting hours start and are with her to the end. At other times she has long conversations with them on her mobile. The other two talk a bit to each other and I lie there listening to their conversations, but don't feel able to join in. I feel more and more cut off and depressed, even at one point almost wishing that I had not survived! But it is not just me feeling depressed. Perhaps any condition affecting the brain makes you prone to depression because every day one or other of my roommates are in tears over something, although this might also be related to the length of time they have to stay in hospital. With Oxford being a regional centre for neurosurgery, like me, they have all been referred here from other hospitals, so their homes are some distance away, and family and friends have to make long journeys to visit. Luckily I don't live so far away, just a twenty mile journey.

But it is now coming up to three weeks since my operation, so I have survived the 'danger period'. That means it should not be long before I will be able to return home once again.

4

Home

'How would you like to go home today?'

It is exactly three weeks since my operation. I have finally had my drip removed and am managing to drink enough to satisfy everyone, just about.

One of the doctors had suggested that I might be well enough to go home a few days earlier, but he had been overruled by one of his seniors, who said I must stay for the full three weeks. Much as I had wanted to go then I had been quite relieved. I was still feeling so helpless; no energy and unable to stay up for more that about twenty minutes before having to lie down again.

Now I admit I am still unsure how I will cope, but am feeling so depressed here that maybe I will be better at home. So I say, yes please, and it is settled.

Lawrie is on his way to visit, so I cannot let him know until he gets here. I start to dress and pack up some of my things ready, and tell him as soon as he arrives. He looks uncertain.

'Are you sure you're well enough?' he asks.

'Well they can't do anything more for me here, so it's just a matter of time for me to get back to normal. I might just as well be at home, that's if you think you can manage. I won't be able to do much for a while.'

He still looks a bit worried, but agrees.

One of the nursing staff comes to see me.

'The doctors have said you can go home today, but you can't go just yet. First we have to get your medication from pharmacy and a physiotherapist needs to check you to see that you can walk on your own. You have your husband to look after you?'

I say yes.

By now I am beginning to feel very tired and nauseated once again. Nausea has become more and more of a problem the last few days. I decide I must lie down again for a bit or I will not have enough energy to be able to cope with the journey. I have no sooner settled down than the physiotherapist arrives and I have to get up again to demonstrate my walking skills. I still have the problem of my balance going every so often and now I am using a walking stick, which I hold in my left hand to steady myself.

'Do you always use a stick?' the physiotherapist asks.

'No. This is just one I sometimes use when I go hill walking. But now I tend to lose my balance a bit and it's always to the left. Having this helps.'

He seems happy with that and says I am alright to go.

I lie down once more, but again not for long. Next a nurse brings me a bag containing my pills with an instruction sheet telling me when they should be taken. She goes over them all explaining when I should take them and that I have to continue the nimodipine for another few days.

She says I can now go.

After all this I really feel exhausted and am torn between resting again for a while and getting home. Getting home wins. Lawrie helps me finish dressing and it feels strange being in my day clothes again. I say goodbye to the others and set off down the corridor. I can't see any nurses around at all, so am unable to say goodbye to them or thank them properly. I haven't seen any of the ones I know today anyway, so they are probably off duty. I have no idea of the way out of the building, and Lawrie leads me to the lift down and out to the car, very close by. We set off.

The journey home, which takes almost an hour, seems endless. I try to look out of the car window, but am unable to focus on anything. Everything looks as if it is rushing past and it is making me feel disorientated. I still have slight double vision when I look to the left, so I try looking the other way, but it is no better. In the end I just look down onto my lap. I discover much later that this feeling of everything rushing past is not uncommon after a subarachnoid haemorrhage, or any other sort of brain injury. What happens when everything is going by so quickly is that the brain is unable to keep up. Trying to concentrate can then just make it seem more muddled. But I do not know anything about this just now and instead think it must be something to do with my double vision.

At last we arrive home. I am feeling awful, even more nauseated, having been up far longer than I have ever managed in hospital. All I want is my bed. As soon as I am in the door I head for the stairs. I put a foot onto the first step—and come to a halt. I have not got the strength to go any further; I cannot lift up my other foot. I lean forward onto my arms to try to pull myself, and with a great effort manage it. But I am still only on the first step.

'I can't get up the stairs,' I wail. Although they had made sure I could walk before leaving hospital, no one seemed to have considered stairs.

Lawrie comes to my aid and pushes me up from behind, one step at a time. It is slow progress. At last I am there and make for my bed, relieved to be able to lie down again and sleep at last.

Now I am home we soon get into a routine. In the morning it is washing and generally sorting myself out. Lawrie has been to the local hardware store and bought a low stool that I can use to sit in the shower. I am very pleased that when we had our new bathroom installed a couple of years earlier we had the foresight to have a grab bar fitted on the wall over the bath, and this is invaluable when I now have to step in, as the shower is over the bath. After all the effort of washing and teeth brushing I am exhausted, so return to bed once again. By tea time in the afternoon I am ready to dress and come downstairs for tea.

On the first day Lawrie comes to help me down the stairs.

'I should be alright going down,' I say.

'Well, I need to stay to make sure.'

It is as well that he does. As I try to step down my supporting leg gives way and I go down heavily onto the first step. I only just manage to stop myself from falling, and might have done if Lawrie had not been there. He helps me down the rest of the way.

'You mustn't ever attempt the stairs unless I am there to help, you promise me,' Lawrie says afterwards. I promise I won't until we are both sure I can do it safely.

After tea he comes with me into the garden, where I walk around slowly, looking to see how much everything has grown while I have been away. It is a lovely sunny day and it feels so good to be outside, but I am soon tired again and we go back in. We sit together in the living room and have our tea Afterwards Lawrie puts on the television, but I can't concentrate on it at all and need to go back to bed.

This is our routine every day for the first week. I think I expected that I would be able to do more once I was home again, but as it is I am almost completely dependent on Lawrie. He brings me my meals in bed. He has never cooked before and I have to explain some things, like the time food needs to be in the microwave. He has bought several packets of ready made fresh soups, and I have either these or a boiled egg (after I have told him how long it needs be boiled) for lunch. He has stocked up on some ready meals and one of our friends has very kindly given us some home cooked pies that just need heating up in the oven, and we have one of these in the evening. I am beginning to eat a bit more now, although have lost a lot of weight—over a stone—during my stay in hospital. I still feel nauseated a lot of the time, but eating helps.

On my third morning home, a Monday, the phone rings at about 9am. I answer, as there is an extension by the bed. It is my GP. She has just got the letter from hospital giving her the details of my stay there. She asks how I am. I tell her I am progressing, if only slowly, and still feel very tired and weak. I go on to say about the nausea and she says she will leave a prescription for me in their reception for Lawrie to collect. This helps, although I still feel nauseated at times. For some reason it is worse when I try to exert myself at all, such as when climbing the stairs.

One thing I have now become more aware of is the tingling in my feet and hands. Only my right hand is affected, and that very slightly, mainly in my index finger, the thumb and middle finger on either side less so. I had not noticed it in hospital, largely because I had my drip in the back of that hand. If I felt any tingling I had thought it was due to not moving it very much for fear of the needle becoming dislodged.

However I am now much more aware of how my feet are affected, especially the right one. It is the top and outer half of each foot where I feel it most, extending up above the outer side of my ankle. It is more altered sensation rather than complete numbness, although a couple of my toes are almost completely numb, and I seem to be hypersensitive to pain and to temperature. Stepping into a warm shower can feel as though it is scalding and has to be done slowly. Sometimes they feel like they are burning hot. At night I often cannot bear even the bedclothes touching them and I end up trying to sleep with my feet over the side of the bed. I also very occasionally feel sudden sharp stabbing pains, although I go for long periods without feeling that at all. None of this really bothers me much though, and most of the time I do not think about it at all. If that is my only long term side effect I think I have done very well.

By the end of my first week at home I am beginning to feel really frustrated that I cannot do more. Lawrie tries to reassure me that I am progressing, and to some extent that is true. I can manage the shower on my own now, but have to go straight back to bed afterwards. When I go downstairs at tea time I am getting little stronger on the stairs, although still need help from Lawrie and I cannot do much else. Lawrie turns on the television to pass the time after tea, but I feel too tired to watch. I try lying down on the settee while I watch, but this does not help. I can barely manage half an hour downstairs before having to return to my bed. When trying to watch television I find cannot take it in at all. It just confuses me, the noise is irritating and I just want to turn it off. In bed I try to listen to the radio. Normally I enjoy Radio 4, but now whenever I try to listen I can't wait for it to be turned off again. Music is no better. I feel better in silence. It sounds boring, but I feel best if I just doze on and off most of the day, and although I am spending most of the day like this I still manage to sleep well at night.

I spite of all this, however, I realize that coming home has been good. Although frustrated by slow progress, my deep depression has gone, partly I think because I do not feel under any pressure to do anything. At times I wonder if I should push myself more to make myself progress, but when I try it just makes me feel awful, so I give in and only do as much as I feel able.

However we still have the problem of the holidays we have booked. We have already had to cancel our trip to France because I was in hospital, and now it is just a week until we are due to go on a short cruise to Ireland. I have been trying to convince myself that it will be restful and I can spend my time sitting back and relaxing, although I won't have the energy to go ashore very far when we are in port. However I now have to admit defeat. I still find that even sitting up for more that about thirty minutes is too much, so I would not even be able to cope with the journey to Southampton to start with. We cancel the holiday.

Our final holiday booked is the most adventurous and the one I have been looking forward to most, not due for over another six weeks. This cruise is aboard a small ship with just fifty passengers in the Arctic, sailing round Svalbard (formerly known as Spitsbergen). There we should be able to see wildlife such as polar bears, walruses and whales in their natural environment. However eventually this has to be cancelled as well because we realise that to enjoy it I would need to be really fit. Also there is the danger that if I am ill again we will be a long way from civilization and specialized medical help. Luckily we are well insured and eventually get all our money back.

Now I have been home for almost two weeks Lawrie thinks it is time to go to see my

GP, and I agree. I am sure nothing more can be done to help my progress and it is just a matter of time, but I know it will reassure Lawrie. He is still so worried about me and I think really it has all been worse for him than for me. He was the one staying with me when I was acutely ill, not knowing if I would survive, visiting me every day in hospital, and now I am home he is the one doing all the work. He rings the surgery for an appointment. Unfortunately my GP is booked up for over two weeks ahead, but he manages to make one for a couple of days ahead with one of the others in the practice, his own GP.

The next day at tea we put on the television. Flicking through the channels I find a program that is just beginning. It is Desperate Housewives. That seems to be about the level I can manage at the moment, so start watching. For the first time I find I actually get engrossed in something and before I realise it the program has come to an end. I have sat there for over an hour. This is a major achievement; I must be getting better at last.

The following day we go together to the GP. He listens as I explain my progress and tell him how slow and frustrating it is, but that yesterday I had felt I might be getting somewhere at last. His comment is that there is probably still some blood in the space around my brain and it will take some time to be fully reabsorbed. Blood is irritating to brain cells and, once it has cleared, I should feel a lot better. This was something I had never thought about, and it makes sense. Both Lawrie and I feel reassured.

Now at last I am beginning to feel my energy is returning and over the next week begin to really make progress. I can soon manage the stairs on my own, taking it slowly and having a pause to rest half way up. I find I cannot push myself too much though, because exertion still brings on the nausea again. One day I do try to see how quickly I can get up stairs, ignoring the nausea, and I do it without a pause, but when I get to the top I have to rush straight to the bathroom where I actually vomit. After that I continue to take things slowly again, pausing as soon as I feel any signs of nausea.

I try to use the computer and start to go through some of the hundreds of emails that have accumulated. This has to done by degrees because each time I try, after a few minutes it gives me a headache.

Several of my friends have been to visit and it is good to see them again. I am able to chat normally at last. For the first time I have the energy to go to the kitchen to make tea or coffee for them. It seems an age since I last did this and I have to think carefully to remember how to do it all.

About six weeks after coming home we need to stock up again on food. Up until now Lawrie has had to do all the shopping on his own. When he goes I feel a bit nervous at being left alone, even though it is not for long. What would happen if I became ill again? This slight nervousness at being alone has never completely left me, even years later. But now I am well enough to join him in the supermarket. It is a task I do not normally enjoy, trawling up and down the endless isles and always remembering something I have forgotten to get on my way home. It is about a six mile drive to get there, and this time I feel fine in the car. Going round the supermarket feels very strange. It is not that I have forgotten exactly, but more as if I have not been there for years and am now remembering it all once again. I feel almost elated, looking at everything on the shelves, and think I should never complain at having to go there again. It is just so good to be able to do it once more.

5

Recovery

Because I have had neurosurgery I am not allowed to drive and I am obliged by law to notify the Driver and Vehicle Licensing Agency (DVLA). I have to await their approval before I can start to drive again, and they will only do this after they have received and reviewed certain information from my surgeon to show that I have been treated and recovered, and do not suffer from any serious after effects, such as seizures, that could make it dangerous for me to drive. The whole process of this review takes months. The hospital has to provide them with the information, and of course the doctors are busy enough without having to do this, so there is a delay. Then the DVLA want more details, by which time it is Christmas, which inevitably leads to further delays. It is mid April, almost a year after my aneurysm burst, that I am finally told I can drive again. After all this time it feels very strange being behind the wheel and I have to concentrate hard on everything I am doing. I feel I have lost my confidence and at times I want to give it up completely, but I cannot leave Lawrie to always have to do all the driving, especially when we go on long journeys—and what would happen if he was ever ill? So I persevere. It takes several months to regain my confidence again.

Once I am able to use the computer again more easily I trawl the internet for more information about the after effects of a subarachnoid haemorrhage. Nobody has ever discussed this with me, although I suppose I have never asked. I find out that some people do have problems with speaking and memory. At first it was sometimes a struggle to find the right words and that was partly why I found talking such an effort when I was in hospital. One of the commonest problems is to use an incorrect word in a sentence, like saying bus instead of car. Occasionally I find myself doing this. I am not sure if it is more frequently than before, because everyone occasionally makes these sort of errors. Maybe I am just more aware of it when I do.

Am I more forgetful? To begin with there were a lot of things that I seemed to have forgotten. For example I had difficulty remembering the names of people that I knew very well, although could usually recall them if I though hard enough. I would also often lose track of a conversation. But what I found rather more strange was that there were times when I was thinking about something and I can only describe it as actually being aware of my thoughts fading. I would try to hang on to whatever I was thinking about, but it would go, and there was nothing I could do about it but hope I would remember again later. After a few months this no longer happened.

Then there is the phenomenon of going upstairs for something and, when there, finding you have forgotten what you have gone up for; something that happens to everyone from time to time. I certainly I do this far more frequently now, but perhaps that is a simply part of getting older.

Another problem I found was that I got dizzy very easily. I belong to a group where we do social dancing, that is traditional formation dances similar to barn dances. Many of the dance movements include turning and, when I took this up again a few months later, I found that turning quickly made me terribly dizzy. I had to avoid such movement. Almost three years later I was surprised to find that I was no longer affected this way and could turn almost normally again. It had taken that long for my brain to recover. I do still find that my balance is slightly affected at times though.

During the first few months of my recovery I felt terribly alone. I know I had my husband, who could not have been more supportive, but he has no medical background. My internet searches gave me plenty of information on subarachnoid haemorrhage and I certainly gained a better understanding. What I did find though was that anything on strokes seem to concentrate almost entirely on ones due to blocked blood supply and tend to ignore subarachnoid haemorrhages.

But what I really would have liked was to have met and talked to someone who had gone through the same thing as me. I have never knowingly met anyone who as recovered from a subarachnoid haemorrhage and I would have loved to have joined a support group, but could not find one. Another option would have been a good on line forum, only again I could not find one at first. Perhaps I did not search hard enough, especially as I could not use the computer for long without getting a headache, but in the end I gave up. However I think the information generally available has improved since then, and eventually I found and joined a good on-line forum that I wish had been available earlier.

Atrial fibrillation.

When an aneurysm bursts most people experience the thunderclap headache, one excruciating explosion as an aneurysm bursts. Mine must have been a rather slower bleed because I heard a long sequence of explosions as the blood pumped out. It was a large bleed, rated 4 on the Fischer scale of 1-4. This sudden influx of blood into the subarachnoid space would have caused an increase in intracranial pressure and amongst other things this pressure can lead to cardiac arrhythmias, that is abnormal and often irregular heart beat.

My heart seemed to stop suddenly as blood was pumped out of the ruptured aneurism and I was not aware of it beating at all for several seconds. Then it slowly started again, but not, it turns out, in a normal rhythm. I was in atrial fibrillation (AF). How do I know this? I know because I have a pacemaker.

A few months after my subarachnoid haemorrhage I went for my routine annual check up in cardiology. Everything that has happened since my previous check up is stored within the pacemaker so that the cardiology technician can see exactly how both the heart and pacemaker are functioning. Apparently my heart was in AF lasting for several hours. I had been attached to a heart monitor when undergoing the coiling operation, and by then I was back in a normal rhythm again, albeit one controlled by the pacemaker, so the AF was not detected. However I did have several further, rather shorter, bouts of AF over the following few weeks.

So what is AF? In a normal heart the atria, the two smaller chambers beat at a steady rate of between about 60-80 a minute. This rhythm is initiated by what is known as the heart's own pacemaker, a small group of specialized cells within the atrial wall. As the atria contract a signal is sent down specially adapted fibres to the ventricles, the two larger and more muscular chambers, stimulating them to contract a fraction of a second later. They pump blood out into the body and this is what is felt when someone takes your pulse rate.

AF is a condition where the atria of the heart beat extremely rapidly and irregularly, so fast that the ventricles cannot keep up. They will only be able to respond to some of the impulses from the atria and the beat will be fast and irregular. The main symptom of AF is thus a rapid and irregular pulse rate. The danger of AF is that, because the atria are not beating normally, some of the blood pools within them and can begin to clot. Some of the clots can then enter the circulation and be carried to the brain leading to a stroke.

In my case, however, I have a pacemaker for heart block. This is where the signals between the atria and ventricles is cut off, either partially or completely. It means that the ventricles beat at their own slower rate, which can be as low as around 30 beats a minute.

A pacemaker works by sending electrical signals from its battery down leads to electrodes implanted in the heart, and these can be set at the desired rate. In my case this is a minimum of 60 beats a minute, (although it is also set up to go faster when necessary). Therefore when I developed AF, none of the signals would have been transmitted to the ventricles, and they just continued to beat at the rate set. My pulse rate would have remained regular and normal, and the atrial fibrillation only detected when I went for a check up later.

I sometimes wonder if the pacemaker saved my life. When my heart stopped the pacemaker would have continued to try to stimulate it to contract and, when in AF, it would have kept the ventricles beating regularly. But that is only my own speculation.

Angiograms.

Six months after going home I return to the hospital for an angiogram. I had one of these when I was first admitted there to diagnose the aneurysm, but have no memory of it at all. The procedure is to insert a tube into my femoral artery and feed this up to my left carotid artery in my neck. From here a radio opaque dye is injected and the scanner records the image as the dye flows along the artery into the brain circulation. In the angiography room I have to lie flat with my head kept completely still, held in position by tape over my forehead. Above me is an array of screens onto which the images will appear. I am told not to try to look at them as it might make me move, but I will be shown them afterwards.

The worst part is having the tube inserted and the doctor needs more than one attempt to get it in, probably due to scarring from earlier times. Once in place they inject the dye. I have been warned that I might feel it and also may see flashing lights, and I do. There is a slight burning sensation behind my left eye and a lot of flashes, which appear as small lines, all at different angles. At the same time the scanner moves from left to right over my head. It is quite close, but again have been assured that it won't touch me and I might find it easier to close my eyes, which I do most of the time. This is repeated two or three times. The burning sensation is more intense on each occasion, but disappears very quickly.

It is soon all over and the tube removed. The main danger now is that I might bleed from where it has been taken out, since it was in an artery. A large wad of dressing is taped over the site to apply a bit of pressure and I have to remain lying flat and keep my leg straight for the next four hours.

Before I am wheeled back to my room I am moved to a position from which I can see the screens where the images from the scans are displayed. They are amazing three dimensional images showing all the blood vessels in different colours, and the images can be rotated so that they can be viewed at all angles. The doctor comes to explain the results and shows me where the aneurysm is, now filled with platinum wire coils. It is so small it is not easy to see at all. Everything looks good he tells me, but there is a bit of the neck of the aneurysm still present and they want to do another angiogram in eighteen months to check it again.

Back in my room I am offered a sandwich lunch, which is the easiest thing to eat lying down, and a drink with a bendy straw. I have a book to read to pass the time. Lying flat makes my back ache again and I am glad when the time is over and I can get up.

Eighteen months later the angiogram is repeated, and now the aneurysm has completely gone. I do not have any more aneurysms, so I do not need any further investigations or treatment. I am cured.

Epilogue

Up to 40% of patients who have a brain aneurysm that ruptures will die, if not immediately then very soon after. I have been one of the lucky ones, making an excellent recovery, for which I am so very grateful. The trouble is that virtually all aneurysms are asymptomatic, so most people never know they have them. But every year a small proportion of these aneurysms will burst, usually without any warning. Even if an unruptured aneurysm is discovered by chance, perhaps as a result of some other investigation, the decision as to whether or not to treat it can be difficult. The treatment, especially if the only option is clipping, which is a more invasive surgical treatment than endovascular coiling, is not without serious risks, such as the aneurysm bursting during the procedure. The question then is, which carries the greatest risk, the surgery or living with the knowledge that you have an aneurysm that has a small chance of bursting at any time.

Looking back, although it seemed devastating at the time, compared to what I have now learnt about other people's experiences with ruptured aneurysms, I think I got through everything fairly lightly. I did develop a degree of vasospasm, but this resolved itself quickly without any serious consequences, and I did not develop any other serious complications as a result of my aneurysm bursting and its treatment. The coiling was successful, no further aneurysms were found and I have made essentially a complete recovery. This recovery has been slow but I followed my instincts and only did as much as I felt able, and my energy returned in its own time. I have learnt that recovery from brain injury cannot be hurried.

Everyone's experience of a subarachnoid haemorrhage is different, depending on the position of the aneurysm as well as the severity of the bleed. My mother's symptoms were very different from mine, with a severe headache and pain down through her neck and back, and she was misdiagnosed at first. This is not an uncommon situation for small bleeds from leaking aneurysms. Many are missed initially, being put down to severe migraines, or to pulled back or neck muscles as in my mother's case. They are then only diagnosed when a more severe haemorrhage ensues, when all too often it is too late.

Why do they develop? No one really knows, although they are more common in people who have high blood pressure or who smoke. There is also sometimes a genetic predisposition, shown by when they are found to run in a family, and since my mother and I both have had aneurysms, my sister has been screened and thankfully found to be clear.

A burst aneurysm is most common during middle age, although they do rarely occur in young adults, often with tragic results. They are virtually unknown in children. Those who survive may go on to suffer from serious complications. Vasoconstriction of the blood vessels to the brain can lead to symptoms of a stroke, although the incidence of this has been reduced considerably since the routine use of nimodipine has been initiated. Some will develop hydrocephalus, an increase in the amount of CSF, which causes pressure on the brain. The treatment is to insert a permanent stent to drain away the excess fluid. Blindness is also not all that uncommon, and this may be permanent due to nerve damage or it can be caused by bleeding within the eye, in which case it can eventually be treated and sight restored. Some may go on to suffer seizures, or are left with other varying degrees of disability, both physical and mental. Also, anyone who has one aneurysm has an increased likelihood of having more, in which case they may need to be treated as well to prevent them rupturing in the future.

I realise how lucky I am to have made such an excellent recovery and am making the most of still being alive. Three and a half years after my aneurysm burst my husband and I have finally been able to go on our cruise to Svalbard, similar to the one we had to cancel when I was ill. It lived up to every one of my expectations. I loved everything there, the wildlife (including polar bears, walruses and whales), the scenery and the remoteness of the Arctic. I am so lucky and thankful that I have been well enough to be able do it at all.

There is a mass of information on subarachnoid haemorrhage and cerebral aneurysms that can be found by a routine online search, therefore I have made no attempt at a comprehensive review. The following are just a few that I have made use of and found helpful. Support groups are a bit more difficult. Although there are plenty of online groups there is little else available for anyone wanting face-to-face contact. Few hospitals are active in this area and initially I found only one. However a couple of years later a new support group was started in Oxford, and this is at the top of the list below.

Head2Head
> https://www.head2headsah.co.uk

This is a focus group for patients from the John Radcliffe Hospital in Oxford. It was started when staff realised the need for support for a patient after their discharge from hospital. Meetings are currently held every three months, but may be increased in the future.

Brain Haemorrhage Support Group
> http://www.bhsupport.org.uk/brainh aemorrhage-699.html

This group gives both online information and holds events and meetings for brain haemorrhage survivors. It is based in Liverpool and was started by an ex-patient of the Walton Centre who experienced the 'sense of abandonment' that so many people feel after their discharge from hospital.

NHS choices

http://www.nhs.uk/conditions/subarachnoid-haemorrhage/pages/introduction.aspx

This site gives basic information and is easy to understand.

Patient.co.uk

http://www.patient.co.uk/doctor/subarachnoid-haemorrhage

This site gives rather more comprehensive detailed information, both for patients and professionals.

Brain & spine foundation

http://www.brainandspine.org.uk/subarachnoid-haemorrhage?gclid=CjwKEAiA5qOlBRDAn8K5qen65joSJADRvlbqo2golY4yPQwbZquY3zam5wkeMB5yalcmvmOhqms4LxoCWcjw_wcB

Information includes a booklet that can be downloaded.

Brain aneurysm foundation

http://www.bafound.org/subarachnoi d-hemorrhage

A lot of detailed information can be found here. It is a US site, so there are some aspects, particularly in after care, that differ from that found in the UK.

Brain Aneurysm Support Community

http://www.bafsupport.org/

This US site has a subgroup for UK members. A very supportive group.

Acknowledgments

Firstly I would like to thank all the doctors, nurses and other staff, without whose expertise I would not have survived this ordeal. Then there is my husband, who gave me endless help and support throughout my illness and recovery, and friends who also gave support.

82944713R00046

Made in the USA
Columbia, SC
07 December 2017